T0144844

BASIC HEALTH PUBLICATIONS USER'S GUIDE

TO STRESS-BUSTING NUTRIENTS

Learn How Vitamins and Other Supplements Can Help You Fight Stress.

ROSEMARIE GIONTA ALFIERI

JACK CHALLEM Series Editor

The information contained in this book is based upon the research and personal and professional experiences of the author. It is not intended as a substitute for consulting with your physician or other healthcare provider. Any attempt to diagnose and treat an illness should be done under the direction of a healthcare professional.

The publisher does not advocate the use of any particular healthcare protocol but believes the information in this book should be available to the public. The publisher and author are not responsible for any adverse effects or consequences resulting from the use of the suggestions, preparations, or procedures discussed in this book. Should the reader have any questions concerning the appropriateness of any procedures or preparations mentioned, the author and the publisher strongly suggest consulting a professional healthcare advisor.

Series Editor: Jack Challem
Editor: Laura Jorstad
Typesetter: Gary A. Rosenberg
Series Cover Designer: Mike Stromberg

Basic Health Publications User's Guides are published by Basic Health Publications, Inc.

CONTENTS

INTRODUCTION

Stress has become an everyday word. Think about how often you or your friends say, "I feel so stressed," or "I've been so stressed out lately." Indeed, stress seems to permeate our lives. How often do you gobble down a sandwich while working at your computer? How much environmental stress do you face on a regular basis, whether from pollution, chemicals, or noise? How stressed out are you because you return from vacation to find 150 e-mails awaiting you? Our overly mechanized, technological society causes a bit of a paradox: The very technologies that purport to save us time and keep us connected can also rob us of peace and downtime.

Do you just have to accept living under constant stress as the price to pay for living in the twenty-first century? Yes, and no. While there is not much you can do to return to a simpler time, there is plenty you can do to help offset the effects of stress and manage it in a healthful way. And how you manage stress may be more important than how much stress you are under. Left unmanaged or mismanaged through bad habits such as smoking or drinking, stress can kill you. Its association with increased risk for disease and death is well known.

The *User's Guide to Stress-Busting Nutrients* focuses on several nutrients that have stress-busting properties and can help you to manage stress in a positive way. They work by providing key biochemical building blocks for the brain, beneficially affecting your mood and nervous system. Some of them, such as selenium, are antioxidants, which, as free-radical scavengers, help prevent stress that occurs at the cellular level. Left unchecked, free-radical damage leads to aging and is associated with increased risk for several diseases including heart disease and cancer.

Other nutrients, such as vitamin C, also work directly on your adrenal system, which goes into high gear during stressful situations, releasing the stress hormones cortisol and adrenaline. These nutrients support the adrenals, helping your body work efficiently to deal with stress.

Still other nutrients, such as zinc, support the functioning of your immune system, which is taxed by stress. Or they treat the various symptoms of stress, including insomnia, depression, and anxiety. Melatonin, for example, is a well-documented natural sleep aid that helps restore your body's natural sleeping cycles, which can become disrupted when you are under stress. There also are several herbs that show promise in offering relief from stress.

Finally, all of us are complicated people with many facets to our lives and personalities. These facets include our relationships with others, our jobs, our spiritual beliefs, and our emotions, among others. If even one of these is off-kilter, it can add to the stress in our lives and increase the amount of suffering we experience. To most effectively deal with stress, we have to look at all of these facets and determine where positive changes can be made. Making small lifestyle changes, such as changes in exercise, in addition to receiving proper nutritional support, can have profound effects on our ability to cope well when under stress.

The *User's Guide to Stress-Busting Nutrients* presents several options for you to consider as you determine which stress-busting approaches are best for you. Remember that we are all unique individuals, with biological, health, emotional, and mental differences that must be taken into consideration when determining the optimal stress treatment program. There is no one-size-fits-all approach to health. As with any health-related program, it is advisable to consult with your healthcare practitioner before taking the supplements or treatments discussed in this guide.

That said, sit back, relax, turn the page, and begin to bust your stress.

CHAPTER 1

ALL ABOUT STRESS

The term *stress* describes any disruption or change in your life (physical, emotional, or psychological) and was first used by Hans Selye, who aptly noted, "Without stress, there would be no life." This is an important point. Many of us identify stress with negative feelings such as worry about our jobs (for example, an author trying to meet a book's deadline, or fear of getting fired) or the negative emotional states that result from relationship issues. Worry, anxiety, fear, anger, depression—these are the feelings we most often associate with stress.

While these all are appropriate examples of stressful situations and states, stress also includes typically happy events such as getting married, purchasing a home, or moving. Your body also experiences physical stress when you catch a cold or suffer from another illness, or even when you suffer from allergies. Toxins in the environment cause stress. Even the hormonal changes you experience throughout your life—from the myriad changes of puberty through menopause—stress your system. In short, any type of change—good or bad—stresses your body.

Essential to Life

So stress is essential to life, which, after all, is all about change. The American Institute of Stress (AIS) notes that good stress, far from being harmful, may actually be beneficial. After all, the positive type of stress results in productivity and can cause us to take action, or to come to new and greater awareness. Think about the nerves of actors before they go on stage. Many actors note that this kind of "nervous energy" is essential for them to give a good performance.

Much in life is like that. The tricky thing is that everyone is different. One person's negative stress may be someone else's invigorating stress. It turns out that the way we perceive stress in our lives is very unique and individualized.

However, there needs to be a proper balance of stress in our lives. As the AIS describes it, stress is like the tension on a violin string. If the string doesn't have enough tension, the sound is dull, while too much tension creates a shrill sound and can even cause the string to break. Even if all the stress you are experiencing falls into the positive category, too much of it may overstress your body and lead to negative physical and/or emotional manifestations. Just the right amount is what is needed—the key is to strike the right balance.

In 1967, the researchers Thomas Holmes and Richard Rahe developed a stress scale, called the Social Readjustment Rating Scale, that assigns values to different life events in terms of how much stress (whether good or bad) they cause. Death of a spouse causes the greatest amount of stress (100 points). Other high-scoring life events include serious personal injury or illness, marriage, retirement, business or work role change, and menopause. As you can see, some of these events are clearly bad, others

Chronic Stress
Habitual stress, which tends to continue over long periods of time. This is differentiated from acute stress, which is stress that is brief in duration.

may be good, and others seem to be neutral. The point is that they all add stress points to your life, and too many stress points equals the potential for problems.

A Modern Epidemic

In 1983 *Time* magazine ran a cover story article that labeled stress "The Epidemic of the Eighties." Twenty years later, the situation seems to have only gotten worse. Stress seems to have become chronic, meaning that it continues over time. In fact, in 1996 *Prevention* magazine found that 75 percent of survey respondents felt that they suffered from great stress one day each week. More and more people are taking antidepressants or are on antianxiety medications and are seeking out other ways to de-stress, such as exercise, yoga, and meditation (more on these positive lifestyle ways to reduce stress in your life appears in Chapter 11).

Experts think that the stress we experience today is more dangerous in many ways because its source is primarily psychological, rather than physical. This is a bit ironic given all the technological advances that on the surface would seem to alleviate psychological stress in our lives, but in reality only keep us constantly connected and "on" twenty-four hours a day, seven days a week.

In older times, most stress resulted from a clear physical danger or threat. For example, a tree falling toward you would elicit a stress response that would include several physical reactions, such as an increase in heart rate and blood pressure to provide more blood to your brain for improved decision making; a rise in blood sugar to provide more energy; the movement of blood to the large muscles of your arms and legs to increase strength and enable you to run away from the danger; and quicker clotting of blood. All these responses would enable you to quickly make the decision that you needed to get away from the tree and would also help you get away faster than normal.

The nature of stress today is more insidious. Modern-day stress stems primarily from such factors as trouble in interpersonal relationships, emotional conflict, and job-related anxiety, and these are all things that don't resolve themselves quickly the way a physical threat does. Think about it: Once you've run away from that falling tree, the stressor is gone and your body can go back to normal. Not so with interpersonal conflict.

As a result, while our bodies produce the same biochemical reaction to stress, that reaction tends to be produced over and over again on a regular basis, making the stress response more a chronic than an acute reaction. This can be dangerous. In other words, the physical changes that are necessary and beneficial in dealing with temporary stress (like the tree falling) can, over long periods of time, increase your risk for a variety of stress-related diseases.

This is an example of a paradox in the way our bodies function: The same thing that can help us, can also hurt us. The term *allostasis* means "maintaining homeostasis or stability through change." In the case of stress, your body tries to right itself by rising to the challenges of a stressful event and responding accordingly. If, however, the response either does not shut down when it is no longer needed, or fails to be activated when it is

Allostatic Load
The state you are in when systems that work to protect your body, such as the stress response, fail to return the body to homeostasis, or balance.

needed, an imbalance will occur. When this happens, it is known as allostatic load.

The Body's Response to Stress

Your body's physiological responses to stress are triggered by the adrenal glands' release of stress hormones, primarily cortisol. When your body faces a stressful event, it undergoes a series of behavioral, neurochemical, and immunological changes. The goal of these changes is to get your body to respond to the stressor and then, ultimately, bring you back to a state of balance (the concept of allostasis). Most experts view the body's reaction to stress as an adaptive mechanism, meaning that it is way the body tries to maintain homeostasis.

Let's take a look at what's behind your body's stress response. It all begins in your brain. When faced with a stressful situation, your brain undergoes a series of reactions that stimulate your pituitary gland to release a hormone called ACTH, which in turn causes your adrenal glands (a pair of small ductless glands that are located above your kidneys) to secrete the stress-related hormones adrenaline and cortisol.

Adrenaline helps keep you alert; it is responsible for increasing your heart rate and blood pressure. You have often heard people say "I got an adrenaline rush" when faced with a challenging task or perhaps a fear-inducing occurrence. This is what they are talking about. An increase in adrenaline production causes your body to increase metabolism of macronutrients (fats, carbohydrates, and proteins) in order to supply you with the energy you need to get out of the stressful situation. As part of this process, your body excretes amino acids and depletes its stores of magnesium in the muscles, as well as calcium.

Cortisol, on the other hand, works slowly as it helps to release energy stores and is vital in preparing your immune system to deal with any threat. Cortisol also helps to protect your body from harmful or pathogenic agents and to contain acquired immune responses, such as allergies or autoimmune disorders. Whatever the cause of your stress—be it physical, emotional, or psychological—cortisol will be secreted in greater-than-normal amounts during a stressful situation.

Because cortisol can suppress the normal functioning of the immune system, it is possible that a stress response, in which cortisol levels stay elevated for long periods of time, can render your body more susceptible to infectious disease. In general, your cortisol levels peak in the early-morning hours and are at their lowest during the night.

The Signs and Symptoms of Stress

There are a variety of signs and symptoms that are associated with stress. These symptoms can be physiological, as well as emotional, psychological, or behavioral. Some of the most common physiological symptoms include hyperventilating, increased heart rate, nervous stomach and indigestion, sweaty hands or perspiring, headaches, sleeping problems, and increased susceptibility to illness.

Emotional symptoms include feelings of anxiety, fear, irritability, and moodiness. Common psychological symptoms are difficulty concentrating, lowered self-esteem, forgetfulness, and worrying. Finally, behavioral manifestations of stress include increased use of negative coping habits such as smoking, taking drugs, and drinking alcohol; loss of appetite or overeating; becoming accident prone; and startling easily.

The Body Breaks Down: Diseases and Conditions Associated with Stress

Several health conditions and diseases are associated with being in a chronic overstressed state. One is the tendency toward being hyperglycemic, or having high levels of blood sugar. The increased production of the hormone cortisol during stressful times produces an increase in the levels of glucose in your body. If this persists, high levels of glucose can lead to type II diabetes, a dangerous and potentially fatal chronic disease that has become all too common in recent years.

In addition to the higher levels of blood sugar, the elevated work of your autonomic nervous system during periods of stress can lead to hypertension, and eventually arteriosclerosis—hardening of the arteries—both of which place you at greater risk for a heart attack or stroke.

In their article "The Response to Stress," Bruce McEwen, Ph.D., and Dean Krahn, M.D., point out that while a stressful situation can initially improve your brain's ability to think and react, being in a chronic stressed-out state can do the opposite. Instead, chronic stress causes atrophy of nerve cells in the part of the brain that controls memory. In addition, the immune system—also initially helped by an acute episode of stress—is damaged or suppressed when under sustained stress, leaving you more susceptible to a host of diseases and conditions.

Related health issues that experts feel are attributable, at least in part, to stress include insomnia, ulcers, anxiety, depression, irritable bowel syndrome, chronic fatigue syndrome (an autoimmune disorder), obesity, chronic pain, cancer, and heart disease. A recent article in the *Journal of the American Medical Association*

(*JAMA*) reported on the results of a study in which 132 patients with coronary artery disease were monitored to determine which factors could trigger the onset of myocardial ischemia, a condition of reduced oxygen and blood flow to the heart. The researchers discovered that mental stress, including tension, frustration, and sadness, more than doubled the risk of myocardial ischemia in the subjects they studied.

Natural Supplements Can Help

What are we to do about all the stress in our lives? After all, if stress is a fact of twenty-first-century life, if it is a byproduct of the way our society functions, is there anything we can really do?

We can be helped by a number of nutritional supplements that work through different mechanisms to reduce the negative effects of stress and can place your body in a fortified position to withstand the onslaught of the modern-day stress army. From the B-complex vitamins, to GABA and taurine, to zinc and lipoic acid, there is loads of help available to you.

A holistic approach to stress, one that involves both behavioral and lifestyle modifications as well as the use of promising supplements, has the potential to help you better manage the stress in your life. Ready to discover which supplements have the most promising stress-busting effects? Let's look at the B vitamins first.

CHAPTER 2

B Vitamins

Vitamins are essential to sustain life. They are tiny compounds that help your body perform the biochemical processes, such as immune function, nutrient breakdown, blood clotting, and hormone support, that enable you to be alive. Not all vitamins are alike. Some, such as A and D, are fat soluble, which means that they are capable of being stored by the body. Others, including the B-complex vitamins, are soluble in water; your body does not have the capacity to store them, and instead excess amounts are excreted within a few days. It is important to replenish water-soluble vitamins frequently to ensure that you do not become deficient.

The B-Team

When we're talking stress, the B-complex vitamins are among the best nutrients you can take to counter its effects. You can think of them as your frontline defense against stress. These vitamins perform a variety of important metabolic functions that include maintaining blood sugar levels as well as maintaining the health of your hair, skin, eyes, circulatory system, and brain function. Many of the B vitamins also are involved in energy production, helping convert fats, proteins, and carbohydrates into energy.

Stress-specific functions of the B-complex vitamins include adrenal gland support, regulation of glucose metabolism, and immune and nervous system support. The B-complex group includes vitamin B_1 (thiamine), vitamin B_2 (riboflavin), vitamin B_3 (niacin, niacinamide, nicotinic acid), vitamin B_5 (pantothenic acid), vitamin B_6 (pyridoxine), and vitamin B_{12} (cyanocobalamin). Of all the B-complex vitamins, B_{12}, B_6, B_5, and B_2 provide the greatest stress-busting properties.

Vitamins B_{12} and B_6 for Nerve Cells and Immune Function

The primary function of vitamin B_{12} is to maintain healthy nerve cells and red blood cells. It also helps to make DNA. Vitamin B_6 is also essential for red blood cell metabolism and for the proper functioning of your nervous and immune systems. When under chronic stress, your immune system is negatively affected. Stress damages the ability of your body to maintain the activity of natural killer cells, which help protect you against viruses and cancers. It also decreases your body's ability to produce secretory IgA, a substance secreted by the body that helps fight disease-causing agents.

Therefore, when under stress, you can certainly use the immune boost that vitamins B_6 and B_{12} provide. In a study conducted by Tokyo University of Agriculture, researchers sought to clarify the role of vitamin B_{12} in immune system support. They studied mice that were deficient in the vitamin and discovered that the immune cells of those mice were compromised. The researchers concluded that vitamin B_{12} plays a role in immune function in mice.

Vitamin B_6 supports your immune system through its role in metabolizing proteins and cellular growth. It also maintains the health of the organs in your body that manufacture white blood cells, which are your body's primary infection fighters. A B_6 deficiency decreases your antibody production and suppresses your immune response.

Your Body's Clock

One of the effects of stress on your body is that it disrupts the natural twenty-four-hour clock (also called circadian rhythm) that schedules the release of hormones, including cortisol, and can affect your sleep patterns. The coenzyme form of vitamin B_{12} (methylcobalamin) can

Circadian Rhythm

The body's twenty-four-hour cycle or schedule for hormone secretion.

help to reset the clock. In his article "Nutritional and Botanical Interventions to Assist with the Adaptation to Stress," Gregory S. Kelly, N.D., notes that supplementation with this coenzyme "might help shift the cortisol secretion peak, helping place the cortisol clock back on schedule." Remember that when you are under stress, your adrenal glands secrete cortisol in large quantities.

In fact, a study reported in *Psychiatry and Clinical Neuroscience* found that treatment with vitamin B_{12}, as well as bright light therapy, helped correct circadian rhythm imbalances connected to sleep disorders.

The Homocysteine Connection

We know that being in a state of stress increases your risk for heart disease and stroke. So does having elevated levels of the amino acid homocysteine. It is possible that homocysteine levels may rise under conditions of stress.

High levels of homocysteine can damage the coronary arteries, which are the walls that transport blood from your heart, making you vulnerable to blockages. Several studies have shown that supplementation with vitamins B_{12} and B_6 can reduce this risk. The *Journal of the American Medical Association* recently reported on the results of a fourteen-year study that followed more than 80,000 women who had had no previous history of cardiovascular disease. Researchers discovered that those women who had higher intakes of vitamin B_6 had lower rates of cardiovascular disease and suggested that this vitamin is important in the primary prevention of coronary heart disease among women. Other studies have shown similar effects for men.

Vitamin B_5—The Stress Star

Of all the B vitamins, it is B_5, pantothenic acid, and most particularly in its active form of pantethine, that is the all-star stress buster. It is often referred to as the antistress vitamin because it enhances the immune system and helps your body withstand stress. This vitamin's primary functions are to manufacture red blood cells and to support your adrenal glands, which, as we've said, go into high gear during stressful events, releasing the hormones adrenaline and cortisol to help you respond to the stressor at hand. It also helps you maintain digestive health and more effectively use other vitamins.

When you are faced with a stressful situation, B_5 is dissipated rather extensively in order to stimulate the release of cortisol. The release of cortisol inhibits your white blood cells (which fight disease) and suppresses your immune response. Vitamin B_5 counteracts this by enhancing your immune system's activity. Remember that even though your body is not responding to a physical threat in most cases of modern-day stress, it still reacts as if that were the case. During times of stress, pantothenic acid helps your adrenal glands by buffering their production of cortisol and other adrenal hormones and enables your body to respond in an efficient and proper way to the stressor.

Russian researchers studied the content of cortisol in the adrenals and blood of rats that were deficient in B_5. They found that just one administration of B_5 in the active form of pantethine improved the adrenal cortex function of the rats.

Sources of Vitamins B_{12} and B_6

The best sources of vitamin B_{12} are animal foods, such as meat, poultry, fish, and milk. You can also obtain this important vitamin through fortified cereals. Because it is found primarily in animal foods, vegetarians are at great risk of having a deficiency of B_{12} and must be vigilant about taking a B_{12} supplement. Others who may have a deficiency include those with an intestinal disorder that limits the ability of their bodies to absorb B_{12}. (Hydrochloric acid in your stomach releases B_{12} from protein during digestion, and it is this stomach acid that separates the vitamin from protein so that it can be absorbed.)

Signs and symptoms of a B_{12} deficiency include weakness, fatigue, nausea, flatulence, and weight loss. Because of the role B_{12} plays in supporting the nervous system, deficiency can also result in neurological changes, difficulty in maintaining balance, confusion, and tingling in the hands and feet.

B_6 can be found both in animal sources— meats, fish, and poultry—and in fruits and vegetable sources such as potatoes, sunflower seeds, walnuts, and tomato juice. While deficiency of B_6 is uncommon in general, older adults tend to have low levels of this vitamin. Symptoms include depression, confusion, and anemia.

Sources of Vitamin B$_5$

Because vitamin B$_5$ is found in all living things (*pantothenic* means "everywhere"), it is easy to find in a number of food sources. The best sources are those that are fresh and not processed. Foods that are highly processed are low in vitamin B$_5$ because the vitamin is depleted during the refinement process. The best sources include brewer's yeast, fresh meats, unprocessed grains, lentils, corn, broccoli, peanuts, sunflower seeds, and salmon, among others.

Most people are not severely deficient in B$_5$ because of its presence in so many foods. In addition, your intestines produce B$_5$. If your diet is high in refined foods, however, you may be at risk for B$_5$ deficiency. If you are deficient in this important antistress nutrient, you most likely will first feel fatigue. Other symptoms of deficiency include depression, loss of nerve function, stomach cramps, difficulty sleeping, and tingling in your hands and feet.

A recommended stress-busting dose of the B-complex vitamins is a compound capsule containing 100 mg of each of the B vitamins with an additional 500 mg of pantothenic acid.

CHAPTER 3

TAURINE, GABA, AND TYROSINE

aurine, GABA, and tyrosine are amino acids that have been found useful as antistress supplements, both in preventing stress levels from getting out of control in the first place and in treating a person when under stress. Before delving into their antistress properties, let's talk a little about the role of amino acids in general.

Your Body's Building Blocks

There are approximately twenty-two nitrogen-containing amino acids. In different combinations, these acids link to form the proteins that are the foundation for all vegetable and animal life. For this reason, amino acids have been called the building blocks of life. Protein is found in your muscles, hair, nails, skin—it is present in every cell of your body—and your body uses it for the growth and repair of all cells.

> **Amino Acids**
> *Known as the building blocks of life, these protein-making organic acids are present in every cell and determine the structure of all living things.*

Amino acids are categorized as either essential or nonessential. Those that are essential are the 20 percent that your body cannot manufacture on its own—you must obtain these through diet or supplements. The majority of amino acids are produced by your liver and are called non-essential. While your body makes these nonessential amino acids, there may be instances, such as when you are under stress, when you do require supplementation.

In addition to forming proteins, amino acids can play important roles in metabolic functions, with some working to ensure proper brain and central nervous system functioning and others acting as neurotransmitters (the chemicals that transmit nerve impulses across nerve cells). This is where the stress-relieving properties of taurine, GABA, and tyrosine come into play.

Neurotransmitter
A chemical substance that transmits impulses across nerve cells. Gamma-aminobutyric acid (GABA) is one of the body's major neurotransmitters.

Taurine—An Abundant Amino Acid

Taurine is found in abundant quantities throughout the body, particularly in the heart (more than 50 percent of the amino acids in the heart is - taurine). It is also found in other muscles, as well as in the brain and central nervous system. In fact, it is the second most abundant muscular amino acid (glutamine is number one). Rather than manufacturing protein, this amino acid instead is found free (it does not link up with others). Taurine acts as a building block for all the other amino acids and has a protective effect on your brain. Levels of taurine are depleted when you are under either physical or emotional stress, causing your body to require more of this supplement during stressful, difficult periods in your life. Low levels of taurine are associated with an increase in anxiety, poor brain function, and seizures. In fact, taurine has been used to treat epilepsy. And experts theorize that a lack of taurine in the developing brain of a child (where it is usually found in concentrations of up to four times greater than in adults) is associated with seizures.

Taurine is referred to as a conditionally essential amino acid, meaning that while your body can manufacture it on its own from cysteine in the liver there are certain times—especially when you are under physical stress or injury—that it cannot make enough to meet your body's demands. Deficiencies of this amino acid are related to a number of conditions, including retinal damage, growth retardation, immunodeficiency, and cardiovascular disorders.

Stress Depletes Taurine

Taurine protects the brain and is useful in treating anxiety, epilepsy, and seizures. The theory is that it can act as a kind of sedative, balancing nerve impulses in the manner of a neurotransmitter. The journal *Brain Development* published the results of a study indicating that a daily oral dose of 750 mg of taurine decreased seizures by more than 30 percent in eleven of thirty-four patients. Those patients who had the highest taurine concentrations showed the greatest response.

In addition to helping alleviate anxiety, there is evidence that taurine increases alertness and improves mood and feelings of well-being. In a placebo-controlled, double-blind study conducted by the Department of Pediatrics at the University of Vienna, scientists studied the effects of an energy drink containing a mixture of taurine, caffeine, and glucuronolactone on the alertness of graduate students. Measurements of the students' motor reaction time, attention, and mood were taken both prior to and following consumption of the drink. Results showed that the students who were given the placebo had decreases in all these areas, while those who drank the mixture did not. The researchers suggested that these effects were due, in part, to the action of taurine in regulating nervous system function.

Protection Against Muscular Injury

You know how important engaging in physical exercise is for the health of your body and mind. But did you know that physical activity—as wonderful as it is for you—is also a great stressor that damages muscle tissue? (If you think about it, the muscular growth that occurs from exercise is a result of tears and damage done and the subsequent repair of tissue.)

Intense exercise is believed to increase the oxidative stress that results from production of free radicals. Free radicals are oxygen atoms that are highly unstable and can do cellular damage. The theory is that left unchecked, such damage can lead to aging and a variety of diseases.

Several studies have shown that taurine is effective in ameliorating oxidative stress. One study, reported in the journal *Amino Acids*, looked at whether muscle levels of taurine were related to the free-radical damage of exercise-induced injury in rats after running ninety minutes on a downhill treadmill. Results indicated that supplementation with taurine increased the levels of the amino acid in the muscles and offered protection from free-radical damage and exercise-induced injury.

GABA—A Powerful Neurotransmitter

The amino acid gamma-aminobutyric acid, or GABA, is created from glutamic acid and vitamin B_6. It is the most prevalent inhibitory neurotransmitter in the nervous system, meaning that it prevents the hyperactivity or overfiring of nerve cells that occurs during periods of high stress and anxiety. You can think of GABA as a shield that blocks messages related to anxiety and stress from reaching your brain's motor centers. Its effect, then, is a calming one. Along with serotonin, it controls levels of depression and anxiety.

In fact, because of its tranquilizing effects, GABA is often used to treat anxiety and depression. A recent issue of the *Archives of General Psychiatry* noted the growing evidence supporting the theory that dysfunction of the GABA systems is associated with major depression. In one study, GABA levels were measured in the brains of depressed patients as well as in a group of people who had no history of mental illness. The results were staggering: The depressed patients exhibited 52 percent lower levels of GABA than the control group. When the GABA system is enhanced, it produces a tonic, calming effect against the adverse stimuli that can bombard you in the many forms of modern life stress.

Tyrosine Fights Depression

Tyrosine is a nonessential amino acid made from another amino acid in your body called phenylalanine. One of its functions is to produce melanin, the pigment that gives your hair and skin its color and that protects your body against ultra-violet light. Your body uses tyrosine to make many brain chemicals such as adrenaline, serotonin, and dopamine that help regulate your moods. If levels of these brain chemicals are off, your mood can be affected, potentially leading to anxiety and/or depression. During periods of chronic stress, the levels of adrenaline become severely affected.

Many experts believe that major symptoms of depression are the result of a deficiency in adrenaline, noting that drugs that deplete the body of adrenaline lead to a decrease in mood and that many of the drugs that are successful in fighting depression act on the adrenaline system. For this reason, deficiencies of tyrosine are associated with depression. Supplementation with tyrosine has had some positive results, although studies to date have been quite small.

One clinical study looked at two patients who had long suffered from depression and for whom MAO inhibitors (drugs commonly prescribed to treat depression) did not work. After taking tyrosine for two weeks at a daily morning dose of 100 mg/kg, both patients showed improvements and were able to lower the dosages of other drugs they were taking for their depression. Another study looked at a thirty-year-old woman who had suffered from depression for two years and who improved after two weeks of treatment with L-tyrosine. However a study that treated outpatients with major depression with 100 mg/kg/day of tyrosine did not find that the amino acid had any positive effects as an antidepressant.

Tyrosine Increases Coping Ability

Tryosine appears to help your body to adapt and cope with stress by reducing the symptoms stress brings on, increasing alertness and arousal, and allowing some people to avoid unpleasant reactions that are typical from stressful situations.

Researchers at Vrije University in Amsterdam studied the effects of tyrosine on sixteen young people. The study participants received 100 mg/kg of tyrosine one day; on another day they received a placebo. On each day, they were asked to perform a series of cognitive tasks that are sensitive to stress while being exposed to a stressor of loud noise. On the days that they took tyrosine, the participants performed better on two cognitive tasks that were highly sensitive to stress, indicating that tyrosine supplementation helped improve thinking ability under stress.

Sources and Dosage

Dietary sources of taurine include animal products such as eggs, meat, milk, and fish; 500–1,500 mg should suffice as a dosage for brain function. Food sources of GABA are meats, fish, and nuts. The recommended dosage for anxiety is 750 mg. Tyrosine is found in chicken, turkey, fish, almonds, soy, milk, cheese, yogurt, and in pumpkin and sesame seeds. A dose of 500–1,000 mg is commonly recommended.

If you are taking MAO inhibitors for depression, you should not take tyrosine because it can cause a severe spike in blood pressure, leading to heart attack or stroke. People who have a history of melanoma also should not take tyrosine.

A word of advice: Amino acids should be taken on an empty stomach, either in the morning or in between meals. Because some amino acids can have toxic effects in high daily doses (more than 6,000 mg), it is wise to proceed with caution and take amino acid supplements in moderation. Taurine is more effective than GABA at crossing the blood–brain barrier (in your brain, capillaries and other cells can prevent absorption of certain substances by the brain, thereby creating a barrier against assimilation). Therefore, taurine taken in supplement form may be more effective than GABA.

CHAPTER 4

ZINC

Zinc is a mineral that is present in nearly all of your body's cells. Minerals are substances that originate in rock formations and are found naturally in the earth. Like vitamins, they act as coenzymes—they are essential catalysts for all of your body's metabolic functions. There are two groups of minerals: bulk minerals and trace minerals.

Your body requires bulk minerals in greater quantities than it needs trace minerals. Zinc is a trace mineral. While you need relatively small amounts of zinc for good health, it is essential nonetheless for many functions. Zinc promotes proper functioning of the prostate gland and growth of reproductive organs, the synthesis of protein, healing of wounds, and a healthy immune system. It is its role in immune system support that is most vital when it comes to discussing zinc as an antistress supplement.

Deficiencies of zinc result in a number of symptoms, some of which include thin, unhealthy nails, growth impairment, impotence, susceptibility to infection, slow wound healing, and frequent colds. Note that diarrhea, kidney disease, and consumption of a lot of fiber can cause your zinc levels to be low.

To better understand zinc's role as an antistress supplement, let's first take a look at how stress affects your immune system.

Stress Busts the Immune System

Your immune system consists of a group of components, including the spleen, tonsils, thymus gland, adenoids, lymph nodes, and white blood cells, that work together to fight infection and protect your body from disease.

When faced with a threat, your body releases cytokines, which act as messengers that go on to stimulate your cells to release compounds that help mediate the immune response. Your im - mune system also protects you from allergies and cancers. A sustained stressful state damages this system and increases your vulnerability to illness. Simply put, stress busts your immune system.

Immune System *The complex system for identifying and attacking foreign substances in the body.*

The National Institutes of Health has reported that people who cared for Alzheimer's disease patients—and who, therefore, are under a tremendous amount of daily stress—had slower wound healing than a control group. Rate of wound healing is an indication of the efficiency of your immune system. Most recently, caregivers for Alzheimer's patients were found to suffer from long-term stress that lasts even years after caring for the patient, and these caregivers are more susceptible to illness.

In addition, in a major article published in the *Journal of the American Medical Association*, researchers provided an overview of the scientific evidence that psychological stress can have negative effects on the immune system response at the cellular level. The authors noted that the hormonal changes resulting from stress cause changes in concentrations of cytokines (also called interleukins). They cite several examples from well-conducted scientific studies of how the body's immune system is compromised by stress. For example, psychological stress can inhibit the response of natural killer cells as well as the production of disease-fighting antibodies.

One study discussed also involved caregivers of patients with Alzheimer's disease, who in this case were matched with noncaregivers; all were given an influenza vaccine. Although all the participants were similar healthwise at the beginning of the study, they differed in response to the vaccine, with the caregivers not getting as much protection from the flu shot. These results indicate that people under chronic stress can suffer from poor immune response to vaccines. By bringing about a poor response to a vaccine, chronic stress can lead to increased risk of illness.

Another study the authors cite, which was published in the *New England Journal of Medicine*, investigated the effects of stress on resistance to upper respiratory tract infections. Subjects completed questionnaires about stress in their lives and were exposed to different strains of colds, then quarantined for days to see if they developed symptoms. Those subjects who indicated higher levels of stress were more likely to develop cold symptoms than those with lower levels of stress.

Zinc to the Rescue

As we've said previously, zinc is a lead player in your immune system. If you are deficient in zinc, you will be much more susceptible to a number of diseases and conditions. Zinc's role in immune system health includes regulating genes within a variety of immune system cells such as the lymphocytes and leukocytes. In addition, zinc enables

Leukocytes
The body's disease-fighting colorless and white blood cells.

the proper development and function of other immune system cells, including the natural killer cells and neutrophils. Finally, deficiencies in zinc are related to improper functioning of the macrophage—an important immune system cell that engulfs and kills threatening organisms.

Lymphocytes
White blood cells, including T cells, B cells, and natural killer cells, that prevent and fight disease.

In fact, all types of immune system cells show a decrease in function when there is a deficiency of zinc. Because zinc acts in so many different ways on the immune system, your susceptibility to a number of disease-causing agents is affected by this mineral.

Even a mild deficiency can produce an imbalance in the functioning of the immune system. The good news is that damage done to the immune cells due to low levels of zinc can be reversed with zinc supplementation.

Anuraj Shankar and Ananda Prasad of the Johns Hopkins University School of Public Health discuss the role of zinc and immune function in an article in the *American Journal of Nutrition*. They note that studies have been conducted on both animals and humans to determine the effects of zinc deficiency and supplementation. These studies show "the essential role of zinc in normal development and function of many key tissues, cells, and effectors of immunity." For example, animals and humans with low levels of zinc have a suppressed immune response and are more likely to come down with illness.

In one study of zinc supplementation that was reported in *Environmental Health Perspectives*, men who received 300 mg of zinc per day for six weeks experienced enhanced immune system functioning.

In another study, Dr. Prasad caused a mildly zinc-deficient state in a group of subjects. At the end of eight to twelve weeks, these people were found to have lower concentrations of zinc in their lymphocytes and decreased activity of the thymulin (a hormone that promotes proper immune function).

And in a trial conducted in India, children age six through thirty-five months were treated for diarrhea with zinc supplements. The children were given skin tests that measured their response to the presence of a variety of infections, including tetanus and tuberculosis, before and after 120 days of zinc supplementation. The children who received zinc had better reactions to the tests. In addition, analysis of the blood cells of the children who received zinc found increases in immune cell strength.

Even if you are not initially deficient in zinc, if you are under prolonged stress, your immune system is compromised. Supplementation with zinc can enhance the working of your immune system, offering protection from stress-induced damage.

There has been some concern about the safety of taking zinc in high doses. Shankar and Prasad point out that while some studies have indicated that high zinc doses can cause anemia, growth retardation, and a depressed immune system, other larger, long-term studies have not shown negative immunological effects from high-dose zinc supplementation. The evidence suggests that high-dose supplementation with zinc over short stressful periods of time is safe, but you should use caution when taking it over the long term.

Relief from Exercise-Induced Stress

If you are someone who enjoys regular, vigorous

workouts that are of high intensity, take note: Athletes who undergo intense training have been associated with a depressed immune function due to the exercise-induced stress the body endures (in particular, the free-radical activity that is a byproduct of oxidation). In an article published in *the Canadian Journal of Applied Physiology,* researchers from the School of Sport and Exercise Sciences of the University of Birmingham reported that it is important for athletes to not only eat a well-balanced diet to meet their high energy requirements, but also take care to get enough zinc as well as antioxidants and B vitamins.

Sources and Dosage

A good place to get your zinc is from the sea: Oysters contain more zinc than any other food. Additional food sources of zinc include brewer's yeast, egg yolks, fish, soybeans, mushrooms, liver, red meat, and poultry. While zinc is found in beans, nuts, and other nonanimal sources, absorption is better with animal proteins. Therefore, the National Institutes of Health advises that vegetarians may need 50 percent more zinc.

The recommended dosages of zinc sup plements for immune system enhancement are 30–50 mg per day and no more than 100 mg. If you take more than 100 mg per day, you will actually be at risk of suppressing your immune system, rather than enhancing it. This is yet another example of how your body needs balance and the proper amount of all nutrients—throw off the balance and what normally does you good can actually do you harm instead.

CHAPTER 5

MAGNESIUM

L ike zinc, magnesium is an essential mineral. However, while your body requires relatively small amounts of zinc (a trace mineral), it needs quite a bit of magnesium (which is a bulk mineral). In fact, magnesium is one of the most abundant minerals in your body, and has been cited as the most important antistress mineral.

Magnesium acts as a catalyst for many of your body's energy-producing functions. It works closely with calcium for many of your body's functions. These two minerals need each other in order to be properly absorbed and used by your body.

As an example, both minerals work to regulate your heartbeat. Your heart muscle is made up of billions of cells and fibers. The fibers that cause your heart to contract are stimulated by calcium and relaxed by magnesium. Therefore, calcium is associated with inducing your heart's—and other muscular—contractions, while magnesium aids in muscle relaxation and regulation of the heart muscle. Magnesium also protects the linings of your arteries from stress when you have a sudden change in blood pressure. Because of the close relationship between calcium and magnesium, it is important to take these minerals in the proper 2:1 ratio of calcium to magnesium.

Magnesium to Relieve Stress

When you are under stress, whether emotional or

physical, your body releases magnesium from your cells. The magnesium is needed both to energize and to calm you during a stressful situation. However, being in a state of chronic stress can deplete your body of magnesium. The higher your levels of stress, the lower your body's levels of magnesium, placing you at risk for deficiency. According to the National Academy of Sciences, nearly 80 percent of Americans may be deficient in magnesium.

If you are deficient in magnesium, you will not experience the positive effects that this mineral has on stress. Deficiencies in magnesium have been associated with increased anxiety and irritability. Other signs of a magnesium deficiency include rapid heartbeat, insomnia, and mental confusion.

In his article "Magnesium: The Stress Reliever," Leo Galland, M.D., notes that type A personalities—those of us who are competitive and highly driven—are more apt to suffer from stress-induced depletion of magnesium than personalities who are less competitive. This is important, because there is an association between people who are type A and an increased risk for heart disease.

Now that you know that magnesium is needed to produce both the energetic response and the calming reaction to stress, let's look at some more evidence of the different ways that this mineral can offset stress.

Magnesium Suppresses the Release of Stress Hormones

There is evidence that magnesium helps to suppress the release of stress hormones. In a study conducted at the Institute of Clinical Medicine, University of Tsukuba, Japan, and reported in the

Canadian Journal of Cardiology, researchers sought to look at the effect of magnesium on adrenaline. For the study, a group of patients were given intravenous infusions of magnesium while a control group received saline. All participants were then given a three-minute handgrip exercise test, which, because it places a person under physical stress, normally results in the release of stress hormones. Interestingly, in the group that received magnesium, levels of adrenaline were not increased by the stress test. This led the researchers to conclude that magnesium can suppress the release of stress hormones by the heart.

Control Group
In a controlled clinical study, a group of people who do not receive the treatment under study. Their results are compared with a group of treated people.

Stress and Blood Pressure

It's no secret that stress increases blood pressure. Studies from a variety of sources show an association between stress and blood pressure. Hans Selye, one of the founding researchers on stress, noted that a stressful event and the subsequent fight-or-flight response cause increases in both heart rate and blood pressure. You've probably heard of white coat high blood pressure—the hypertension that people with normal blood pressure experience because they are nervous at the moment that their doctor takes their blood pressure.

If you are under chronic stress, your blood pressure can become chronically elevated—and this has serious implications for your health. High blood pressure causes your heart to go into overdrive to pump blood through your body. The many conditions that are caused at least in part by high blood pressure include hardening of the arteries, heart disease, stroke, kidney disease, and congestive heart failure.

Until recently, blood pressure under 140/90 was considered normal. However, research has shown that even lower levels can place you at greater risk for cardiovascular disease, stroke, and heart attack. This evidence has caused the medical community to now consider blood pressure readings of above 120/80 as prehypertension, meaning that while you may not have high blood pressure, you are likely to develop high blood pressure at some point in the future.

Magnesium Lowers Blood Pressure

There is good scientific evidence that magnesium supplementation can help lower blood pressure. In 1998, the journal *Hypertension* reported on a study conducted by Japanese researchers at the Division of Hypertension and Nephrology at the National Cardiovascular Center in Osaka. The researchers studied sixty patients, men and women age thirty-three to seventy-four, who had blood pressures greater than 140/90 over two eight-week periods; they were given magnesium supplementation for one of the two periods. This was a crossover study, meaning that for half the study period, each group received treatment. At the end of the study, researchers found that blood pressure was significantly lower during the period of magnesium supplementation. The authors concluded that "magnesium supplementation lowers blood pressure in hypertensive subjects and this effect is greater in subjects with higher blood pressure."

In another study also reported in *Hypertension*, researchers from the Department of Nutrition, Harvard School of Public Health, looked at the relationship between nutrition and hypertension in more than 40,000 women nurses between the ages of thirty-eight and sixty-three. The women completed nutritional questionnaires at the beginning of the four-year study. Results indicated that those women who did not come down with hypertension during the course of the study were more likely to have consumed magnesium and fiber, as well as a diet rich in fruits and vegetables.

Sources and Dosage

Sources of magnesium are varied. Much of our magnesium comes from drinking water. In addition, it is found in dairy products, meat, fish, seafood, a variety of fruits, green leafy vegetables, nuts, tofu, and whole grains.

Many calcium/magnesium supplements contain 800 mg calcium and 400–450 mg of magnesium. While these are the standard recommended dietary allowances for these minerals, because of the high prevalence of magnesium deficiency, some experts have begun to recommend an increased intake in magnesium to as high as 1,200 mg/day and a change in the ratio of calcium to magnesium from 2:1 to equal amounts of these two minerals.

CHAPTER 6

VITAMIN C

If vitamins belonged to a kingdom, vitamin C (also called ascorbic acid) would most likely be king, so varied and necessary are the functions it performs for your body. Included among the many roles of this powerful vitamin are the production of collagen for muscles and blood vessels, wound healing, and enhancement of your immune system.

Vitamin C is one of your body's strongest antioxidants and as such offers protection from a variety of diseases. Antioxidants are substances that fight the damage posed by free radicals in the cells of your body. Normally an atom contains a balance of paired electrons, which encircle the nucleus. Free radicals are atoms or molecules in which at least one electron is un - paired, causing an unstable envi-

Antioxidant
A substance that scavenges free radicals in the body, preventing them from doing damage.

ronment. This unstable environment enables the electrons to be very reactive, and they can easily bond with other molecules. This process can cause damage through oxidation.

While it is normal for free radicals to occur in the body as byproducts of many metabolic functions, when present in large amounts, they can wreak havoc on your DNA as well as cause muscular and cellular damage. This cumulative damage leaves you more vulnerable to a host of diseases, including heart disease and cancer. Because the effects of free-radical damage build up over time, it is thought to be responsible for most of the symptoms and conditions related to aging.

Vitamin C to De-Stress

When it comes to protection against the damaging effects of stress, vitamin C is an essential nutrient. First, because of its antioxidant properties, it can fight the free-radical damage wrought by a variety of stressors, including those that are physical, environmental, and emotional in origin. In addition, when you are under stress, vitamin C assists your adrenal glands in the regulation of stress hormones.

This increased activity can lead to depletion of the vitamin as it is excreted through the urine. As a water-soluble vitamin, vitamin C cannot be stored by your body; it instead is excreted—making supplementation a must. The white blood cells of people under stress, including smokers (smoking places your body under increased stress), have a decreased ability to retain vitamin C. So it becomes particularly important to take extra vitamin C when you are under increased psychological, emotional, or environmental stress. Let's look at some of the evidence.

Vitamin C Reduces Blood Pressure, Cortisol Levels, and Feelings of Stress

Recently, researchers at the University of Trier in Germany, noting that high doses of ascorbic acid had reduced stress in laboratory animals, decided to conduct a study of the effects of ascorbic supplementation on stress in human beings. The researchers note that prior to their study there was some indication of vitamin C's potential to relieve stress in humans. In particular, they men-tion one uncontrolled trial of elderly women with coronary heart disease who received 1,000 mg of ascorbic acid and 200 mg of vitamin E. These women experienced improvements in immunity and reduced levels of cortisol.

The Trier clinical trial, which was reported in the journal *Psychopharmacology*, was a randomized, double-blind, placebo-controlled study, making it highly scientific and valid. Of the 120 healthy young people studied over fourteen days, 60 were given 3,000 mg of vitamin C each day and 60 were given a placebo.

All were subjected to acute psychological stress in the form of public speaking and having to complete arithmetic mentally. They were asked to rate their levels of stress on a scale from 0 (no stress) to 10 (worst stress). In addition, because stress increases blood pressure and cortisol secretion, participants' blood pressure and cortisol levels were measured. At the end of the study, the group that received vitamin C experienced lower increases in blood pressure, experienced fewer feelings of stress, and had a faster return to normal (prestress) cortisol levels than those in the control group who did not receive the vitamin.

While the researchers could not tell exactly why the stress-protective effects occurred, they speculated that ascorbic acid supplementation could help to regulate stress-related transmission of nerve cells in the brain and that ascorbic acid produces antistress effects. In the end, they concluded that "treatment with high-dose sustained-release ascorbic acid palliates blood pressure, cortisol and subjective response to acute psychological stress."

Vitamin C Puts the Brakes on Adrenals

Scientists have also explored the possibility that

ascorbic acid can actually have a braking effect on the release of stress hormones such as cortisol. In other words, they've looked at whether increased intake of vitamin C can lower the amount of cortisol that the adrenals need to release in response to stress, thereby decreasing the drain on your body.

A study reported in the *Journal of Nutrition* indicated the possibility that this is so. Forty-two male guinea pigs were randomly assigned to a variety of groups and given differing amounts of ascorbic acid. The researchers found that the pigs given higher levels of ascorbic acid had lower levels of activity in the adrenals, leading them to suggest that a megadose of ascorbic acid can inhibit the production of cortisol from the adrenals.

Human studies on this braking effect of vitamin C are hard to come by. However, the *International Journal of Sports Medicine* published the results of a study conducted on ultramarathon runners, who are under a great deal of physical stress. Forty-five participants in a 90-kilometer marathon were studied. They were divided into three equal groups of fifteen participants. For a total of ten days beginning one week before the race, one group received 500 mg a day of vitamin C, another group 1,500 mg a day of vitamin C, and the third a placebo. Blood tests taken immediately after the race revealed that levels of cortisol were significantly lower in the group that took 1,500 mg of vitamin C than in the other two groups, as were adrenaline levels. This study indicates that supplementation with higher doses of vitamin C can lower the release of adrenal stress hormones.

Vitamin C Protects Your Skin

You might not think of your time spent lying on a beach as stressful; in fact, you probably think it is pure relaxation. While that may be the case for your mind and emotions, the hours spent exposed to sunlight present a significant environmental stress on your body. As a powerful antioxidant, vitamin C prevents damage done to the skin by exposure to the ultraviolet rays of the sun.

In a study reported in the *British Journal of Dermatology*, researchers studied the effectiveness of antioxidants in protecting skin against sun damage. The study participants had vitamin E, melatonin, and vitamin C applied to their skin thirty minutes before being exposed to ultraviolet rays. Results showed a protective effect from the vitamins.

Vitamin C Prevents Damage Caused by Oxidative Stress

Oxidative stress occurs when free radicals are formed. As we've already mentioned, free radicals occur in all living things, and are a natural byproduct of cellular activity. The most common free radical in humans is an oxygen radical, which occurs in the mitochondria when an unpaired electron interacts with oxygen. The mitochondria are our cells' power plants, the tiny structures that provide energy for all our life functions. When free radicals are formed in the mitochondria, they reduce the power of the mitochondria to produce energy efficiently. Worse yet, they often damage DNA in the mitochondria as well as proteins and fats. As previously noted, this damage leads to a variety of debilitating diseases and conditions.

Vitamin C can prevent the dangerous changes to DNA that are caused by oxidative stress. Researchers at Memorial Sloan-Kettering Cancer Center in New York City recently studied the role of vitamin C in maintaining the integrity of genes and discovered that cells loaded with vitamin C experienced a significant decrease in damaging mutations or changes. They concluded that the study's findings supported the theory that vitamin C in high concentrations can prevent oxidation-induced mutation in cells.

As we've mentioned previously, while physical exercise is recommended by health experts and considered essential for good health and fitness, long-term vigorous activity can place stress on the body, releasing a significant number of free radicals. A study conducted at the Universitat des les Illes Balears in Spain looked at the effects of vitamin C supplementation on red blood cell antioxidant enzymes during athletic competition and after recovery. For the study, sixteen athletes were divided into two groups. One group received vitamin C supplements; the other acted as a control group. Those in the group that received the vitamin C supplements had better levels of red blood cell antioxidant activity, indicating that vitamin C supplementation can play a role in defending against oxidative stress caused by exercise.

In another example of vitamin C's protective effects, a study reported in the *Journal of the American Medical Association* found that high levels of ascorbic acid were associated with low levels of toxic lead in the blood. The cross-sectional study looked at 4,213 youths and 15,365 adults who had had no history of lead poisoning. It found that those with the highest blood levels of ascorbic acid had an 89 percent decreased prevalence of elevated blood lead levels compared with those who had the lowest levels of vitamin C.

Cross-Sectional Study
A scientific study that looks at a specific group to determine the presence or prevalence of a condition at a given time.

Sources and Dosage

Your body does not produce any vitamin C; you must receive it exclusively through a diet that is high in fruits and vegetables. Foods with high levels of this vitamin include grapefruit, strawberries, broccoli, tomatoes, spinach, blueberries, and green peppers. The vitamin content of these foods is greatest when they are eaten raw or only lightly cooked. Organ meats are also good sources.

Vitamin C deficiency is rare today, but remember that when under stress, your body places great demands on vitamin C, making extra supplementation a wise idea.

Vitamin C supplements are available in tablet, capsule, and chewable forms. An esterified form of vitamin C is also available. Your body may be able to maintain esterified C in your blood cells for longer periods of time than standard vitamin C. In addition, if you find that vitamin C upsets your stomach or if you take aspirin regularly, you may want to try esterified C, which tends to be a bit gentler on the digestive system. Esterified C is formed when vitamin C reacts with a particular mineral, such as potassium or zinc. In addition, esterified C enters your blood and tissues four times faster than regular forms of the vitamin.

Esterify

To convert to an ester, an organic compound formed by a process that neutralizes acids.

Experts recommend dosages of between 500 and 1,500 mg a day. Because vitamin C must be replaced frequently, it is best to take supplements with meals two or three times a day. While studies have found that vitamin C is safe in relatively large amounts (up to 1 gram a day), taking more than 2,000 mg a day increases your chance of upset stomach.

CHAPTER 7

SELENIUM

Stress busting and selenium go hand in hand. This vital trace metal, which is a component of many proteins, acts as an antioxidant that protects cells against free-radical damage resulting from excessive stress. It also supports your immune system and plays a role in sperm mobility and fertility. Selenium is an essential trace mineral found in plant foods grown in selenium-rich soil.

Antioxidant Protection

As an antioxidant, selenium works with vitamin E to combat the stress caused by the oxidation of fats. Fats are oxidized (combined chemically with oxygen) during athletic activity. This can lead to an increase in free radical production. A study reported in the *Journal of the American College of Nutrition* looked at the effects of giving selenium and other antioxidant supplements to athletes to see if the stress (and subsequent release of free radicals) that results from vigorous sustained activity could be lessened.

In the study, a group of triathletes were given 150 mcg of selenium, 2,000 IU of retinol (vitamin A), 120 mg of ascorbic acid, and 30 IU of vitamin E in the form of alpha-tocopherol. Analysis of their blood plasma revealed that after taking the supplements, the athletes had a better, reinforced response to the exercise, with lower levels of exercise-induced oxidative stress.

There is also evidence that oxidative stress from free radicals can increase risk of heart disease. Selenium acts in concert with fellow antioxidant vitamin E to maintain a healthy heart. In fact, low levels of selenium have been associated with heart disease.

In a study conducted at Erasmus University Medical School in the Netherlands and reported in the *Journal of the American Medical Association,* researchers examined the association between selenium levels and risk of heart attack by comparing both the selenium levels and the amount of activity of glutathione peroxidase—an enzyme that is formed by the protein glutathione and selenium—in eighty-four people who had suffered heart attacks and eighty-four healthy people who served as controls.

Results indicated that members of the study group had lower levels of selenium in their toenails than those in the control group. Selenium levels in the toenails are a reflection of how much selenium has been in the blood for up to a full year before the sample is taken. Therefore, low selenium in the toenails could mean that those in the study group had had low selenium levels in their blood before having had heart attacks. In addition, those who suffered from heart attacks demonstrated higher activity of the enzyme glutathione peroxidase, which indicates that the body was trying to defend itself against increased oxidant stress.

While this study makes a good case for selenium's protective effects on the heart, experts warn that additional, larger controlled studies need to be conducted.

Selenium Strengthens the Immune System

We know that chronic stress has a negative effect

on your body's immune system. Selenium plays a large role in immune system support, with low levels associated with damage to white blood cells and the thymus. The thymus gland is the major immune system gland; it sits in between your thyroid gland and your heart and produces your immune system's T cells, a type of white blood cell that fights infections as well as cancer and autoimmune disorders such as allergies and arthritis.

By supporting the thymus, selenium gives your immune system a protective boost. Elevated levels of selenium have been associated with a reduced risk of cancer and inflammation. It also is thought to be helpful for HIV-positive people, helping delay the onset of AIDS—an immune deficiency disease—by energizing the immune system and preventing oxidative stress.

Experts also note that selenium-deficient animals have been found to have lower T-cell blood counts and an impaired ability to produce active white blood cells. They also are more apt to fall prey to infections.

In a review of the research on selenium and immunity that was published in *Environmental Research*, selenium was found to influence all aspects of the immune system. The authors found that deficiencies lead to suppression of the immune system—mainly by harming the body's ability to resist infection and to produce lymphocytes. On the other hand, supplementation with low doses can enhance or restore immune system function by stimulating neutrophils (those white cells that engage in phagocytosis, attacking and destroying tumors and bacteria).

Phagocytosis
The process by which white blood cells attack and kill tumors and bacteria.

More Is Better

When it comes to selenium, it looks like more is better. Research indicates that it may be helpful to take supplements of selenium even if your levels are not initially low. Consider the results of one randomized controlled study, conducted at the New York University Dental Center, in which patients who had at least the recommended levels of selenium were given either a placebo or 200 mcg of selenium each day for eight weeks. At the end of the study, the natural killer cell activity of the group that took selenium had increased by 82.3 percent since the beginning of the study. Natural killer cells are your body's main defense in preventing the development of cancer. In addition, overall lymphocyte ability to kill tumor cells increased in this group.

Researchers attributed this immune system enhancement to selenium's ability to increase the number and type of white blood cells that destroy tumor cells. The results led the researchers to conclude that because of its ability to enhance the immune system, people should take supplements of selenium even if they are getting adequate amounts in their diets.

Despite this strong evidence for the immune-enhancing effects of selenium, there have been studies with conflicting results. In one such study, forty Finnish people all from a group with low levels of selenium received either supplements of selenium or a placebo for eleven weeks. When the study period was over, the group that re - ceived selenium showed slightly higher activity of the immune system killer cells that fight bacteria, but the changes were not significant.

The Cancer Connection

Because selenium can increase the activity of

natural killer cells, which are vital in stopping the formation of cancer in your body, it may be helpful in the prevention of cancer—a disease considered to be caused at least in part by sustained environmental and/or emotional and physical stress. In the process of phagocytosis, natural killer cells destroy cells that have become cancerous, preventing their spread throughout the body.

The *Journal of the American Medical Association* reported the results of a recent study conducted by the Arizona Cancer Center at the University of Arizona. In the study, researchers sought to find out if nutritional supplements of selenium would decrease the number of new cancer cases in people who had already had skin cancer. This randomized, placebo-controlled, double-blind study, which was conducted at several locations, looked at a total of 1,312 patients ranging in age from eighteen to eighty who had a history of basal cell or squamous cell skin cancers. One group was given 200 mcg of selenium a day; the other, a placebo. The researchers wanted to see if the group that received selen-ium would have fewer future cases of skin cancer, as well as any other type of cancer.

The results of the study were a little surprising. While selenium treatment did not really influence whether a person came down with skin cancer, it significantly reduced the risk of getting and dying from all types of cancers combined. The study's authors concluded that while selenium supplementation did not protect against development of skin cancer, it may have reduced the risk of getting and dying from several other cancers, including those of the lung, colon, and prostate.

Food Sources and Dosage

Selenium is found primarily in plant foods. It is also found in some meats, especially in areas where animals eat grains from soil that is rich in selenium. Brazil nuts are particularly high in selenium, with 1 ounce containing 840 mcg. Other good sources include brewer's yeast, walnuts, tuna, turkey, broccoli, brown rice, wheat germ, and whole grains.

While selenium can be found in a variety of food sources, the amount actually present in a given food depends upon the selenium content in the soil that a particular plant grew in. You may think you are eating a food with a high selenium content, but depending upon where it was originally grown, the same food can vary significantly in the actual amount of selenium it contains. In the United States, soil in Nebraska and North and South Dakota is very high in selenium. Countries such as Finland have low levels of selenium in their soil, and their populations are at risk of being deficient in this mineral.

People with nonfunctioning digestive systems who must receive nutrients through an IV line absolutely must take supplements of selenium. Other gastrointestinal disorders can also hurt your body's ability to absorb selenium. Symptoms of selenium deficiency include exhaustion, infections, sterility, and high levels of cholesterol. Deficiency of this mineral has been linked not only to a depressed immune system, but to cancer and heart disease, as well.

Experts suggest a dosage of about 200–400 mcg a day of selenium. Taking more than 400 mcg can lead to excessive selenium in your system and a toxic condition known as selenosis.

CHAPTER 8

ALPHA-LIPOIC ACID

Alpha-lipoic acid is receiving a lot of attention these days for its energy-enhancing and antiaging capabilities. As an energy producer, alpha-lipoic acid helps convert macronutrients (fats, carbohydrates, and proteins) into energy in the mitochondria—the tiny parts of your cells that manufacture the fuel, which supports your energy needs.

Alpha-Lipoic Acid for Stress Busting

Alpha-lipoic acid is a good stress-busting nutrient. When you are under periods of prolonged stress, you feel drained and lack the energy to get through even the simplest of daily tasks, which suddenly seem daunting. You can see how supporting your body's energy system, which is overly taxed during extended periods of stress, would be useful.

In addition, this fatty acid coenzyme is an extremely potent antioxidant that scavenges the dangerous free radicals we produce when under stress. It also reinforces the antioxidant abilities of vitamins C and E and the amino acid glutathione. Alpha-lipoic acid's power as an antioxidant lies in the fact that it is both fat and water soluble, and able to work at the cellular level to combat oxidative stress.

Alpha-Lipoic Acid Improves
Insulin Resistance

Insulin resistance is a condition characterized by the body's inability to process glucose with normal levels of insulin, resulting in an increased production of the hormone. This condition often is the result of a diet that is too high in refined carbohydrates such as white rice, pasta, and white bread. Left unattended, insulin resistance leads to diabetes, a potentially deadly disease that has become an epidemic in the United States.

You may not think of diabetes as a stress-related condition, but increased oxidative stress plays a role in the formation of this disease. Health practitioners in Germany have been using alpha-lipoic acid for more than twenty years to treat diabetes, in particular the peripheral nerve damage associated with the disease. When blood sugar levels are left uncontrolled, eventually diabetics will lose sensation in their feet, and the nerves that supply internal organs will be damaged. Treating diabetics with alpha-lipoic acid can reduce oxidative stress, improve insulin sensitivity and nerve blood flow, and slow down the progression of cell damage.

A study conducted at the University of Heidelberg, Germany, looked at 107 patients with diabetes. Those who received 600 mg a day of alpha-lipoic acid for more than three months had lower levels of oxidative stress and greater antioxidant defense. Another study, conducted by the Mayo Foundation in Minnesota, looked at whether treatment with lipoic acid could reduce oxidative stress in the peripheral nerves of diabetics. The researchers treated diabetic rats with varying dosages of lipoic acid. After one month, these rats showed reduced effects of oxidative stress.

In addition, insulin resistance is prevalent in people who have been diagnosed with depression—a common condition for people under great stress. Researchers have theorized that insulin levels and activity play a role in the proper functioning of serotonin, a compound that is associated with mood levels and our sense of well-being. They believe that depressed people can be helped with alpha-lipoic acid because of its ability to increase insulin sensitivity.

Alpha-Lipoic Acid Fights Effects of Toxins

Alpha-lipoic acid can help protect against the damage caused by such environmental stresses as radiation, smoking, and heavy metal poisoning. *Free Radical Biology and Medicine* reports that treatment with lipoic acid can reduce oxidative damage and help organs function normally in people who have been exposed to radiation. In fact, children living near the Chernobyl nuclear accident site in the former Soviet Union have been successfully treated with lipoic acid.

Alpha-Lipoic Acid Treats Burning Mouth Syndrome

Burning mouth syndrome is a condition char-acterized by severe pain in the mouth. It is considered to be a disease of the nervous system brought on by stress because the pain is not associated with any other underlying physical problem and often has psychological roots. Experts believe that it may be related to the production of free radicals released during stressful situations.

Burning Mouth Syndrome
A condition char-acterized by severe mouth pain, which is thought to be brought on by stress.

In fact, a study conducted in Sweden's Nordic

School of Public Health found that women suffering from burning mouth syndrome were likely to be concerned about the meaning of life and to be under psychological and social stress.

In addition, researchers at the University of Medicine and Surgery in Naples, Italy, conducted a double-blind, controlled study on sixty patients with burning mouth syndrome. They found that the majority of those treated with alpha-lipoic acid showed a significant improvement in symptoms after two months of treatment.

Alpha-Lipoic Acid Prevents Hypertension

In an interesting new finding, it appears that alpha-lipoic acid treatment can also prevent high blood pressure, as well as high blood sugar. The *American Journal of Hypertension* reported the results of a study that investigated whether supplementation with lipoic acid could prevent oxidative stress in the heart and the development of hypertension and insulin resistance.

For the study, rats were given either an alpha-lipoic-acid-supplemented diet or their normal diet. All rats were given high levels of glucose, which would normally increase blood sugar levels. Those that received the supplemented diet experienced only small rises in blood pressure, oxidative stress, and blood sugar resulting from the increased glucose consumption. The authors concluded that alpha-lipoic acid supplementation prevents development of hypertension and hyperglycemia by preventing an increase in oxidative stress.

The promising results of this study suggest the need for further study in humans.

Food Sources and Dosage

Alpha-lipoic acid is found most abundantly in red

meats, particularly in heart muscle and liver. Other sources include spinach, brewer's yeast, and wheat germ. While your body normally can produce all the alpha-lipoic acid it requires, under periods of high stress you may need supplementation. This is especially true if you are a vegetarian.

Supplements are available in capsules and tablets. While the ideal dose is not known, a daily dose of about 50 mg is often advised.

CHAPTER 9

MELATONIN

Like a precious gemstone, sleep has become increasingly rare. With so much else to do in a technological society that functions 24/7, sleep often takes a backseat to all else, leaving us to yawn and caffeinate ourselves as we sleepwalk through each day. For many of us, it is very difficult to get the seven or eight hours of sleep each night that health experts deem essential for our well-being.

And that's during normal times, when things are going well. Imagine when you're under increased stress. It comes as no surprise that stressful events can cause people to have difficulty falling and staying asleep. Most likely you've experienced this at some point in your life. You have a deadline approaching at work and you find yourself tossing in the middle of the night, unable to release troubling thoughts about getting the job done on time. Or relationship problems are depriving you of a restful night. According to the National Sleep Foundation, an independent nonprofit organization dedicated to improving public health and safety by achieving understanding of sleep and sleep disorders, "emotional stress is a major cause of why people can't sleep."

Sleep after Trauma

Stress experienced as a result of a traumatic or

catastrophic event can have a particularly negative effect on quality of sleep. This type of stress is known as post-traumatic stress disorder and is diagnosed when a person who has undergone a severely traumatic event, such as surviving a natural disaster, has psychological symptoms that persist over time.

Most of the scientific studies conducted to investigate the nature of sleep disturbances in people with post-traumatic stress involve small groups of victims of a variety of events including accidents, natural disasters, and violent attack. In several of these studies, survivors experienced disturbances in sleep. One study looked at the survivors of the Oklahoma City bombing and found that 70 percent experienced insomnia six months after the attack; 50 percent suffered from nightmares. Nightmares often involved a reliving of the event. Female victims of post-traumatic stress seem to suffer from sleep disturbances more frequently than men, a fact not surprising given that sleep-related problems are more common in women in general.

Post-Traumatic Stress Disorder
A disorder resulting from exposure to a highly stressful event, such as a natural disaster or accident.

Interestingly, research indicates that when faced with a traumatic event over a sustained period of time—for example, Londoners during the bombing blitz of World War II—people learn to adapt and are able to sleep fairly well.

Insomnia Stresses You Out

In addition to resulting from chronic or traumatic stress, insomnia can actually cause your body to become stressed. Think about how you feel when you've gone a few days on only a few hours of sleep each night. You're more irritable, easily agitated, have difficulty concentrating, and are more prone to emotional upset—all symptoms of overstress. In fact, if you suffer from insomnia you are at higher risk for depression, anxiety, and substance use. Unfortunately, the prevalence of insomnia has increased in recent years.

Sleep deprivation is a serious national problem. Researchers have found a strong association between sleep disorders and illness. The National Institutes of Health estimates that 50 million to 70 million Americans suffer from sleep-related disorders or problems, with a major impact on the ability to function, as well as on physical and mental health. In recognition of the seriousness of this issue, the NIH has released the 2003 Revised National Sleep Disorders Research Plan, which urgently calls for increased study of insomnia as well as the development of therapies, including complementary and alternative medicine therapies, for insomnia of all types.

Melatonin to the Rescue

Enter melatonin, a hormone that is secreted by your brain's pea-sized pineal gland. Hormones are compounds secreted by the endocrine glands, which regulate many of your body's functions. For example, they regulate your reproductive system and sex drive, your growth, and your moods. Melatonin is a hormone made by the neurotransmitter serotonin; its primary function is to synchronize the timing for the secretion of hormones.

Hormone
A substance, secreted by the endocrine glands, that regulates a variety of bodily functions.

Your body releases hormones according to a circadian rhythm, which is the natural twenty-four-hour cycle for biological processes. Think of your body's release of hormones as being set by an inner body clock. At specific and different times each day, your body releases particular hormones to receptive organs or tissues.

In addition to overseeing the overall timing of hormone secretions, melatonin affects how awake or asleep you feel. Melatonin is produced during the dark of night in order to regulate your body's natural clock. When your melatonin levels rise, you feel sleepy; when they drop, you feel more awake. For this reason, melatonin often is referred to as the sleep hormone, and supplements have been used to induce sleep and offer relief from jet lag. The hormone also has been called "nature's nightcap."

Several studies conducted on melatonin show promise for its use as a sleep aid, something that will come in handy if you find yourself suffering from stress-induced sleeplessness. While there are other pharmacological sleep aids available for insomnia, they come with several possible side effects including feelings of drowsiness the following day, loss of memory, and difficulty functioning—not exactly what you are looking for from a sleep aid. In addition, there is the potential to develop a dependency on prescription sleep aids if they are used for long periods of time.

Nature's Sleep Aid

A study conducted by researchers at Oregon Health Sciences University and reported in the *New England Journal of Medicine* tested melatonin's effects on a group of blind people. Blind people were selected for the study because their inability to distinguish light and dark cycles makes them more vulnerable to sleep problems.

In the study, participants were given 10 mg of melatonin or a placebo each day, one hour before they went to bed. Researchers found that when given melatonin, the participants' body clocks returned to the normal twenty-four-hour cycle, while the participants slept for longer periods of time and felt more rested and alert the next day. The study's authors noted that melatonin could also help people who aren't blind develop more normalized sleep patterns but warned that the proper dose and time to take melatonin might depend on the type of sleep disorder.

In another study, volunteers were given varying small oral doses of melatonin (0.3 or 1.0 mg) or a placebo in the evening hours. Researchers then measured the time it took to fall asleep, to reach stage two in sleep, and to reach rapid eye movement (REM) sleep. When they took melatonin at either dose, the volunteers fell asleep more quickly and entered the deeper stage two sleep more quickly. In addition, melatonin did not delay the onset of REM sleep. In other words, melatonin helped improve both the quantity and quality of sleep. Furthermore, none of the study participants experienced negative effects, such as drowsiness or headache, as a result of taking melatonin. The researchers concluded that taking oral supplements of melatonin before sleep can treat insomnia.

Several studies have revealed that administering melatonin in oral dosages of as little as 0.3 mg is sufficient to promote and sustain sleep in insomniacs. Melatonin has been found especially useful in fighting insomnia experienced by older adults, whose natural melatonin levels have dropped as part of the aging process.

Melatonin and Stress Reduction

Undergoing a surgical procedure places great stress on your body, with corresponding sharp rises in stress hormones. An interesting study conducted by researchers in Cairo and reported in the *English Journal of Anesthesiology* investigated melatonin's effect on the release of stress hormones due to surgery. The researchers looked at eighty male and female patients between the ages of nineteen and fifty who were to undergo surgery. Some patients randomly received small doses of melatonin prior to surgery. Before and after surgery, blood levels of cortisol and adrenaline were recorded.

The results of this study indicated that melatonin was effective in reducing the stress response in individuals undergoing surgery, and in possibly protecting the body against stress-induced damage. It seems that melatonin produces this effect by enhancing your body's production of endorphins, which are neurochemicals that relieve pain and reduce anxiety. In addition, heart rate and blood pressure were reduced in the patients who took melatonin.

Finally, melatonin is effective in reducing oxidative stress in your body by acting as a strong antioxidant. Melatonin protects the nucleus of your cells, which is the central part of the cell that contains genetic materials, against the damage done by free radicals. It does this both by killing free radicals and enhancing the antioxidant properties of other compounds. In addition, melatonin stimulates the transport of electrons and the production of energy in the mitochondria.

While the above-mentioned studies indicate melatonin's usefulness in combating insomnia, the National Sleep Foundation cautions that more research in the area is needed.

Dosage Recommendation

Melatonin supplements should be taken at night, approximately thirty minutes before going to bed in order to correspond with your body's natural rise in melatonin during the night. While this hormone appears to be safe at the recommended dosages, note that the commonly recommended dose of 3 mg per day is greater than the levels of melatonin that occur in your body naturally. This high dose has the potential to affect your body's circadian rhythms and could trigger grogginess, drowsiness, and nightmares.

For this reason it is wise to limit daily supplementation to 0.1 mg to 0.3 mg. You can start with the lower dose and increase if need be.

If you are pregnant or nursing, you should not take melatonin, since there is not enough information on potential effects of the hormone to a fetus or infant. In addition, people with severe allergies or autoimmune disease should avoid melatonin supplementation.

You also can try to maintain high melatonin levels by eating regularly, eating lightly at night, avoiding stimulants such as caffeine, and avoiding vigorous exercise close to bedtime.

CHAPTER 10

HELPFUL HERBS

Several herbs can also help your body deal with the negative effects of stress. The healing and medicinal properties of plants are well known. Botanicals have been used by different cultures to both prevent and treat diseases and conditions for centuries.

That said, there are cases of unsubstantiated claims, and because herbs are very potent medicines, there is valid concern over the wisdom of taking herbs blindly for any condition, including stress. This does not mean you should be afraid of herbal remedies. You do, however, need to be an educated, aware consumer.

Read up on the herbal treatments that you are considering taking and examine the results of studies as well as the anecdotal folk medicine history of a particular herb. In addition, and perhaps most important, always discuss any herbs you are considering with your doctor or primary healthcare practitioner. Together, you can determine if there are any potential negative interactions with other medications you may be taking, as well as the herbal treatments that will best meet your own unique biological needs.

While you may have read or heard media reports about the controversy surrounding herbal remedies, in particular with regard to their potential toxicity and effectiveness, when used correctly, and under the supervision of a health practitioner, herbs can be safe and very effective natural medicines. While there are many herbs that can help you de-stress, in this chapter we'll look at ginseng, kava and valerian, and St. John's wort— a few of the most commonly prescribed herbs to combat stress.

Ginseng—A Powerful Adaptogen

A class of herbs called adaptogens is considered extremely helpful for stressed-out people. Adaptogens help your body deal with the stress caused by environmental conditions such as heat, cold, and exposure to toxins, as well as with stress that is emotional or psychological in nature. In addition, they enhance the immune system and support your adrenal system. By helping to bring your system back into a state of balance (which, when under stress, it is far from), they also provide an energy boost.

Adaptogen
A substance that helps the body adapt to environmental, physical, or emotional stress.

Ginseng is considered one of the strongest adaptogens around. This herb, which has been used as a medicine in the Far East for several thousand years, comes in a variety of forms. The Asian variety is called *Panax ginseng*. Another common form is American ginseng, which is very similar in chemical makeup with some slight variations. Be aware that another common and inexpensive herb known as Siberian ginseng is, in fact, not really part of the ginseng family and does not have as strong a reputation as an adaptogen as the real ginsengs.

Studies performed on animals have shown that injecting them with *Panax ginseng* offered protection against toxins such as radiation, improved mental function, and protected against exhaustion and stress. Other studies have looked at oral doses of ginseng and found that the herb can increase endurance during periods of extreme stress. Human studies have found that *Panax ginseng* can stimulate the immune system and improve a person's mood and mental state.

Ginseng Improves Your Mental State

When you are under stress, you can feel like your mind is going. You are easily confused, you forget things, you can't focus. Researchers from the Human Cognitive Neuroscience Unit at Northumbria University in the United Kingdom report that recent research has shown that even a single dose of *Panax ginseng* can improve memory.

In addition, the *Natural Health Bible* reports the results of one study in which 112 middle-age adults were given either ginseng or a placebo over two months. Those who received the ginseng experienced improvements in their abstract thinking. Interestingly, though, in other areas of mental function, such as memory and concentration, there was no significant difference between the two groups. More controlled clinical studies on ginseng's effects in this area are warranted.

Safety and Dosage

In a scientific review article in *Public Health Nutrition,* experts discuss the safety of ginseng. They note that while ginseng has been a popular herbal remedy for a long time and while there is evidence that it can be taken safely and effectively, there is a need for additional randomized, double-blind, placebo studies. That said, studies in animals have indicated that use is nontoxic.

The recommended dose of *Panax ginseng* is 1–2 g of the herb, or 200 mg of extract. *Panax ginseng* is quite expensive, so beware of lower-priced supplements, as they are likely impure and contain other substances such as caffeine.

Valerian and Kava to Soothe Nerves

Among the most common symptoms of stress are anxiety, nervousness, and difficulty sleeping. Valerian and kava are nervines, herbs that have a calming and sedating effect on the body and can be used to alleviate agitation and nervousness during times of stress.

Nervine
A category of herbs that support the nervous system, which is compromised under stress.

The root of valerian is used for medicinal purposes, most commonly as a sleep aid. Experts believe that valerian may work by affecting the amino acid GABA. You'll remember that GABA is a powerful neurotransmitter that helps keep you in a calm state. Valerian works in ways that are similar to the commonly prescribed tranquilizer Valium.

Kava, which comes from the pepper family, has a long history of use among Pacific Islanders, who mixed the herb with coconut milk as a beverage for social occasions and ceremonies. This herb was traditionally known for its mild intoxicating effect. In addition, one of its active ingredients is kavalactone, a sedativelike substance, which makes this herb useful for the treatment of anxiety. In fact, clinical studies indicate that people given kava exhibit fewer symptoms of anxiety, such as nervousness, heart palpitations, restlessness, and chest pain.

Better Sleep and Response to Stress

Kava and valerian have been found to be useful sleep aids, providing a restful night's sleep without creating a dependency or causing significant side effects. In a study published in the journal

Human Psychopharmacology, patients who were suffering from insomnia caused by stress were treated with 120 mg of kava for six weeks. Afterward, they were taken off treatment for two weeks and then given 600 mg a day of valerian for six weeks. Finally, after another two weeks off treatment, they were given a combined treatment of kava and valerian for six weeks.

The study measured stress in terms of social, personal, and life events. Results indicated that total stress was relieved by both valerian and kava taken individually as well as when taken in combination. Side effects, including dizziness and vivid dreams, were minor, with most participants experiencing no side effects at all.

In addition to helping you get a good night's sleep, these two herbs have been found helpful in reducing some of your body's physical reactions to stress. Researchers at the University of Surrey in the United Kingdom looked at whether kava and valerian could offset the effects of psychological stress. In this study, fifty-four people, divided into three groups, performed a color/word mental stress task twice within a week's time period—once before receiving treatment, and once after.

Following the first test, two groups were given kava or valerian for one week, while the third group served as the control. The blood pressures and heart rates of participants were measured as indicators of stress both before and after the stress task. Results showed that the groups that took either valerian or kava had drops in systolic blood pressure and felt less mental pressure when performing the stress task after having taken the treatment. In addition, the group taking valerian had lower heart rates in reaction to stress.

Kava Controversy

In July 2002, the Food and Drug Administration (FDA) issued an advisory alerting consumers that the use of kava carries potential risk of severe liver damage, including hepatitis, cirrhosis, and liver failure. The advisory was based on reports from health authorities in several countries.

However, in a related article published on www.healthy.net, Hyla Cass, M.D., notes that the majority of the reported cases of liver damage involved people who took kava at the same time they were taking other drugs that are toxic to the liver, including some prescription antianxiety medications, or alcohol. Bear in mind that even pain relievers containing acetaminophen, such as Tylenol, can cause liver damage when taken by people who drink alcohol regularly. Cass points out that a review of seven clinical trials published in 2000 in the *Journal of Clinical Psychopharmacology* found that kava was effective and safe in relieving symptoms of anxiety, without significant reports of liver damage.

In general, experts agree that more investigation into kava's safety and efficacy is warranted. For now, the recommendation of the American Botanical Council is that anyone who has any liver problems, is taking a drug that has adverse effects on the liver, or regularly drinks alcohol should not take kava.

Dosage Recommendations

The recommended dosage for insomnia is 2–3 g of valerian as a dried herb or 270–450 mg of extract in water about an hour before going to sleep. For kava, the recommended dosage is 210 mg of kavalactones, also taken an hour before bedtime. For anxiety relief, take 2–3 g of valerian twice a day and 40–70 mg of kavalactones three times a day. Do not take more than 300 mg of kavalactones in a given day. Note: While found generally quite safe, a downside to valerian is its strong odor, which many people find bothersome.

St. John's Wort for Depression

Depression is a medical condition with biological, psychological, and social causes. Symptoms include a persistent sad mood, loss of energy, difficulty concentrating, feeling worthless, sleeping too much or having difficulty sleeping, and loss of interest in what previously gave you joy.

Gone are the days when people were thought to be able to just snap out of a depressed state or mood. The medical community now recognizes this often debilitating condition as a real and serious medical problem that requires treatment and is often genetically based. Stress can trigger bouts of depression in people, especially in those who are genetically predisposed toward it. In fact, scientists have recently found that people with a certain type of gene in their brains are more apt to suffer from depression after a stressful event or trauma.

St. John's wort, *Hypericum perforatum,* is a yellow flowering plant containing chemical compounds that have been used for more than 2,000 years to treat a variety of conditions, most notably depression. In Germany, St. John's wort has been the medicine of choice for depression for years. The theory is that St. John's wort prevents nerve cells in your brain from reabsorbing the neurotransmitter serotonin, which greatly affects your mental state. It also may play a role in the functioning of your immune system.

Studies indicate that St. John's wort is useful for treating mild to moderate depression. The

British Medical Journal in 1996 published a review of twenty-three studies, which indicated that St. John's wort was effective in treating depression without as many side effects as commonly prescribed antidepressants.

However, one large recent study, commissioned by the National Institutes of Health, found that St. John's wort was no more effective than a placebo in treating major depression of moderate severity. This study involved 340 participants at various sites and was conducted in two phases. The study measured the number of people whose depression improved with St. John's wort compared to those given the commonly prescribed pharmaceutical sertraline (the drug Zoloft). A third group was given a placebo.

The study found that 24 percent of those taking St. John's wort responded to the treatment, which—while statistically about the same as for a placebo—was also similar to the response to sertraline. This is important because it showed that the overall response to sertaraline was not better than the response to St. John's wort. The researchers attributed this to the fact that such results, in which response to a placebo is similar to response to treatment, are not uncommon in trials of even approved antidepressants.

Dosage Recommendations

While St. John's wort has been safely taken by many people for many years, it can have negative interactions with certain drugs, in particular drugs used to treat HIV-positive people and certain chemotherapeutic drugs, making those drugs less effective. The most common side effects of St. John's wort are dry mouth, dizziness, gas - trointestinal symptoms, sensitivity to light, and fatigue. As with all herbal medicines, make sure to discuss with your doctor all other medications you are currently taking if you plan to take St. John's wort.

How to Take Herbs

When taking herbs, buy brands that are reputable and contain pure ingredients. Those that are organic are best. Look for standardized extracts of medicinal plants, which means that the product has been analyzed to ensure that it contains certain vital components. In addition, tinctures (alcoholic extracts of plants) and freeze-dried extracts are considered more stable and concentrated, making them the preferable form in which to take herbs. Never suddenly go off a prescribed medication to take an herbal one; this can lead to severe withdrawal that may be life threatening

Stop taking an herbal treatment if you notice any kind of allergic reaction, and make sure you report any such reaction to your doctor. Because herbs are very potent medicines—after all, they are forms of natural drugs and are not foods or vitamins—take them cautiously. Remember that all of us are biologically and emotionally different. While a particular herb at a certain dosage may be good for one person, it may not necessarily be helpful, and may be harmful, to another.

CHAPTER 11

LIFESTYLE APPROACHES

The supplements and herbs discussed in this book can help you to reduce or manage the effects of stress in your life. In addition, it is vital to take a look at your whole life and approach stress management in a holistic way that recognizes and honors your physical, emotional, mental, and spiritual sides. Like equal slices of a circle, you cannot be whole if any of those parts is missing or incomplete. All require attention. This chapter addresses some of the changes you can make in your behavior and thinking to help you deal with stress positively, as well as recommended lifestyle changes that will keep your body fortified against stress.

Coping Strategies

Stress contributes to bad health both through the physical toll it takes on your body as well as through the unhealthy habits that people commonly acquire when under stress. Let's look at these first. Scientists talk about the ways we manage stress as our coping strategies. Whether we know it or not, when faced with stress we employ ways to cope. These strategies run the spectrum from maladaptive such as denial, avoidance, engaging in alcohol or drug abuse, or overeating to positive coping strategies such as reframing a situation, positive self-talk, and engaging in relaxation techniques like yoga and meditation.

If you find that you cope with stressful experiences by doing something negative—such as smoking or drinking—you are using a strategy that may artificially calm you down in the short run, but is in fact only contributing more layers of stress. Most likely, engaging in this kind of coping strategy results from avoiding or denying that the stress exists.

For example, people will drink alcohol thinking that because alcohol has sedative effects it will calm them down. However, alcohol is also a depressant. It can lead to worsening of mood. In addition, the chemicals in alcohol stress your body at the cellular level, wreaking damage to organs such as the liver.

To cope positively with stress, you first need to appraise the stressful situation—to determine how significant and controllable a stressful event is, as well as to assess how you can deal with that event. Often when we are feeling overwhelmed, we have a distorted conception of how much control we have. When you appraise the situation, ask yourself the following questions: *Can I change the situation? If not, can I manage the way I react emotionally? Do I believe that I can make it through a stressful situation successfully?*

This belief that one can successfully manage a stressful situation, which social scientists refer to as self-efficacy, has been studied and shown to be instrumental in your actual ability to overcome adversity. Think about the classic children's story *The Little Engine That Could*. The engine believed it could carry the cars full of toys over the mountain even though it had never done anything like that before—and it did, in fact, succeed, largely because it thought it could.

Self-Efficacy
A person's internal belief in his or her ability to succeed at something.

Action and Thought

Social researchers have come up with a widely recognized model for coping with stress, called the Transactional Model. This model organizes the way you can cope with stress into two broad categories: One is problem management; the other, emotional regulation. Problem management addresses what you actually do to reduce the stress or to deal with it. On the other hand, emotional regulation refers to how you can alter the way you think or feel about the stress. In other words, this model looks at both how you can act and how you can think in ways to reduce stress.

Examples of problem-focused management are seeking more information about a particular stressor so that you feel more educated and in control, as well as taking active steps to reduce the stress. As an example, if you are under great stress because your boss at work is driving you crazy, on your case all the time, your problem-solving strategy might be to actively engage in a job search.

Examples of emotional regulation or management include expressing your feelings, looking at the stressful situation in a different way, and seeking social support from friends, family, or professionals. To use the same situation of the difficult boss, you might discuss the way you are feeling with some family or friends, who may be able to help you to see that perhaps your boss is dealing with other work- or home-related issues that are spilling over into his or her management style with you. This may help you not to take your boss's short temper personally.

While there may be no way to actually rid yourself of a stressor, the way you perceive the stress and your ability to have some control over its effects can determine whether or not stress will become something you can manage, or something that will manage you.

Now that we've discussed your mental and emotional approaches to stress, let's turn to some of the lifestyle changes you can make to deal more effectively with stress.

Manage Your Time

One of the common reasons people cite for being stressed today is lack of time to accomplish all that life demands of us. You have what seems like three days' worth of tasks to do in a single day. If you work on how you manage your time, you will find that your stress level most likely will take a nosedive.

The first step in managing your time is to develop priorities: Make a list of the things that you need to do on a given day, then rank each of those tasks in descending order, with the most important listed first. Be proud and content with accomplishing the two or three most important goals. The others can wait until tomorrow.

Try to analyze your dead time—how much time do you spend on mindless television watching, for example? Find those spots in your day during which you might be able to do something more productive and more satisfying.

Remember that you can only do your best given time constraints and all your obligations and responsibilities. You do not have to be perfect. No one is.

Actively Relax

The opposite of stress is relaxation. In fact, the body's responses to both stress and relaxation are as different as laughing and crying. The stress response includes an increase in heart rate, blood being moved away from the skin and most organs, and an increase in sweat production.

The relaxation response instead is marked by reduced heart rate and blood pressure, movement of blood toward your internal organs, and a decrease in the production of sweat. The term *relaxation response* was developed by Harvard researcher Herbert Benson. Benson believed that you could actively bring about the beneficial calming effects of the relaxation response by engaging in relaxation techniques.

You may wonder how on earth this can be possible if you are in such a nervous or agitated state to begin with. The fact is that you can learn techniques to relax your body and your mind. Just by engaging in these techniques, you train your body to experience the physical effects of relaxation by calling upon the parasympathetic nervous system, which controls bodily functions during periods of rest and relaxation.

Deep Breathing to Relax

One of the most popular and simple relaxation techniques is deep breathing. In this technique, instead of breathing shallowly through your chest, you focus on using your diaphragm. Inhale deeply through your nose, drawing your breath from the base of your lungs. Imagine that you are filling up your lungs as if they are balloons. Take four or five full seconds to inhale. Then exhale slowly, taking at least the same amount of time—if not longer—to exhale. Repeat the breaths ten times. This simple technique will lower your heart rate and replace states of anxiety with calm.

Relaxation Response *Physiological responses that are the opposite of those caused by stress.*

Other Relaxation Techniques

There are several other ways you can bring about

the relaxation response. The ones you select depend upon your own inclinations—what feels right to you, what you enjoy, what is consistent with your spiritual beliefs, and so forth. Some of the most popular are prayer, meditation, massage, yoga, and visualization.

Another interesting technique may be especially helpful to people who constantly worry. Try setting aside half an hour during the day as your "worry time." For that half hour, you can worry all you want, but then you are not allowed to worry at any other time during the day. This technique helps reduce anxiety in chronic worriers who may otherwise spend large portions of their day in an agitated state.

Eat Well and Exercise

This seems obvious, but it's amazing how when we are stressed out we often tend to eat poorly (bingeing on junk "comfort" food, for instance) which only increases the stress state. For example, if you tend to fill up on refined carbohydrates and simple sugars, you are at risk for glucose intolerance, which has been linked to depression. Or if stress leads you to drink more coffee to feel alert, you may in fact be increasing your anxiety levels. And if alcohol is what you turn to in the belief that it will calm you down, you are in fact increasing the stress on your body and disturbing your sleep cycles.

Instead, eat a healthful diet that is rich in nutrient-dense foods—the good fats such as omega-3 fatty acids found in fatty fish and olive oil; complex carbohydrates such as brown rice; and plenty of lean protein, vegetables, and fruits. Set aside time for your meals; don't gulp them down in a rush. Try to envision mealtime as a well-deserved opportunity to relax and unwind.

Finally, regular exercise also has a stress-busting effect. Even though your body initially experiences physical stress due to exercise, over time it adapts to the stress demand and reaps several antistress benefits. Exercise, especially aerobic exercise, releases naturally occurring opiates in the brain, which help us feel positive. Research has shown that people who regularly exercise are less apt to be depressed, tense, or worried. If you are new to exercising, you don't have to do a lot. Try a thirty-minute brisk walk (about fifteen minutes per mile) four or five times a week.

Seek Help

Finally, if you find that your efforts to reduce stress in your life don't seem to be working and that you are living in a nearly constant state of stress and anxiety, it may be time to consult a professional. Ask your health practitioner or a friend to recommend a therapist, or contact a spiritual adviser who may be able to guide you through a stressful period and work with you on finding the treatment approaches that will work for you.

CONCLUSION

S tress is a fact of life. As we live, we experience stress. Both the natural and expected
changes that occur in our lives on a daily basis, as
well as those that are unexpected, are stressors.
Not all stressors are equal. Some events, such as
the loss of a loved one, add tremendous stress to
our lives; others only minimally affect us.

In and of itself stress is not bad. Some stress is,
in fact, good. It is necessary. It prompts us to act,
to be creative, to have that burst of energy to
achieve goals. Much like actors who take the
stage every night depending upon those butter-
flies in the stomach to give them the inspiration
to deliver their best performance, good stress
makes us productive.

You've seen how your body is equipped to
handle stress. It has remarkable systems in place
to remove you safely from a threatening situation. Ideally, after a stressful situation your body
goes back to a state of balance. It is when stress
becomes chronic and unmanageable, when your
body cannot revert to that equilibrium, that stress
becomes dangerous.

To manage stress, it is best to take a holistic
approach that looks at the way you are living your
life in all areas—emotionally, physically, mentally,
and spiritually. Simple lifestyle changes that
affect these areas can have a great impact on
your ability to handle or reduce stress. In addi-

tion, many nutritional supplements, particularly those discussed in this guide, can help you minimize stress so that you have energy, peace, and a positive outlook.

Managing stress is a lifelong endeavor. The nature of the stressors will vary at different times in our lives. At times they will be work related, at other times relationship or health oriented. Whatever their cause, there is no need to feel you are a victim of stress. This guide has shown you there is much you can do to combat stress and live life to its fullest.

SELECTED
REFERENCES

Abu-Zeid H, Samahan Y, Omar S, et al. Efficacy of melatonin premedication on the stress response to intubation and surgery: comparative study with midazolam and clonidine. *English Journal of Anesthesiology*, 2002; 18:99–105.

Anisamn H, Merali Z. Understanding stress: characteristics and caveats. *Alcohol Research & Health*, 1999; 23(4):241–250.

Brody S, Preut R, Schommer K, et al. A randomized controlled trial of high dose ascorbic acid for reduction of blood pressure, cortisol, and subjective responses to psychological stress. *Psychopharmacology*, 2002; 159(3):319–324.

Clark LC, Combs GF, Turnbull EH, et al. Effects of selenium supplementation for cancer prevention in patients with carcinoma of the skin. *Journal of the American Medical Association*, 1996; 276(24):1957–1963.

Glaser R, Rabin B, Chesney M, et al. Stress induced immunomodulation: implications for infectious diseases? *Journal of the American Medical Association*, 1999; 281:2268–2270.

Gullette EC, Blumenthal JA, Babyak M, et al. Effects of mental stress on myocardial ischemia during daily life. *Journal of the American Medical Association*, 1997; 277(19):1521.

Kelly GS. Nutritional and botanical interventions to assist with the adaptation to stress. *Alternative Medicine Review*, 1999; 4(4):249–265.

Kiremidjian-Schumacher L, Roy M, Wishe HI, et al. Supplementation with selenium and human immune cell functions II. Effect on cytotoxic lymphocytes and natural killer cells. *Biological Trace Element Research*, 1994; 41(1–2):115–117.

Midaoui AE, Elimadi A, Wu L, et al. Lipoic acid prevents hypertension, hyperglycemia, and the increase in heart mitochondrial superoxide production. *American Journal of Hypertension*, 2003; 16(3): 173–179.

Ohtsuka S, Oyake Y, Seo Y, et al. Magnesium sulphate infusion suppresses the cardiac release of noradrenaline during a handgrip stress test. *Canadian Journal of Cardiology*, 2002; 18(2):133–140.

Rimm EB, Willett WC, Hu FB, et al. Folate and vitamin B_6 from diet and supplements in relation to risk of coronary heart disease among women. *Journal of the American Medical Association*, 1998; 279(5): 359–364.

Sack RL, Brandes RW, Kendall AR, et al. Entertainment of free-running circadian rhythms by melatonin in blind people. *New England Journal of Medicine*, 2000; 343(15):1070–1077.

Sanacora G, Mason GF, Rothman DL, et al. Reduced cortical gamma-aminobutyric acid levels in depressed patients determined by proton magnetic resonance spectroscopy. *Archives of General Psychiatry*, 1999; 56(11):1043–1047.

Seidl R, Peyrl A, Nicham R, et al. A taurine and caffeine-containing drink stimulates cognitive performance and well-being. *Amino Acids*, 2000; 19(3–4): 635–642.

Shankar AH, Prasad AS. Zinc and immune function: the biological basis of altered resistance to infection. *American Journal of Clinical Nutrition*, 1998; 68 (suppl):447S–463S.

Wheatley D. Stress induced insomnia treated with kava and valerian: singly and in combination. *Human Psychopharmacology*, 2001; 16(4):353–356.

OTHER BOOKS AND RESOURCES

Balch PA and Balch. *Prescription for Nutritional Healing*, third edition, New York, New York: Avery, 2000.

Barney P. *Doctor's Guide to Natural Medicine*, Pleasant Grove, Utah: Woodland Publishing Inc., 1998.

Challem J and Brown L. *User's Guide to Vitamins and Minerals*, North Bergen, New Jersey: Basic Health Publications, 2002.

Glanz K, Marcus Lewis F, Rimer B (editors). *Health Behavior and Health Education*, second edition, San Francisco, California: Jossey-Bass, 1997.

GreatLife Magazine
Consumer magazine with articles on vitamins, minerals, herbs, and foods.
Available for free at many health and natural food stores.

Let's Live Magazine
Consumer magazine with emphasis on the health benefits of vitamins, minerals, and herbs.

Customer service:
1-800-676-4333
P.O. Box 74908
Los Angeles, CA 90004

Subscriptions: 12 issues per year, $19.95 in the U.S.; $31.95 outside the U.S.

Physical Magazine

Magazine oriented to body builders and other serious athletes.

Customer service:

1-800-676-4333

P.O. Box 74908

Los Angeles, CA 90004

Subscriptions: 12 issues per year, $19.95 in the U.S.; $31.95 outside the U.S.

The Nutrition Reporter™ newsletter

Monthly newsletter that summarizes recent medical research on vitamins, minerals, and herbs.

Customer service:

P.O. Box 30246

Tucson, AZ 85751-0246

e-mail: jack@thenutritionreporter.com

www.nutritionreporter.com

Subscriptions: 12 issues per year, $26 in the U.S.; $32 U.S. or $48 CNC for Canada; $38 for other countries.

INDEX

Printed in the USA
CPSIA information can be obtained
at www.ICGtesting.com
JSHW051957150824
68134JS00050B/90